Table of Contents

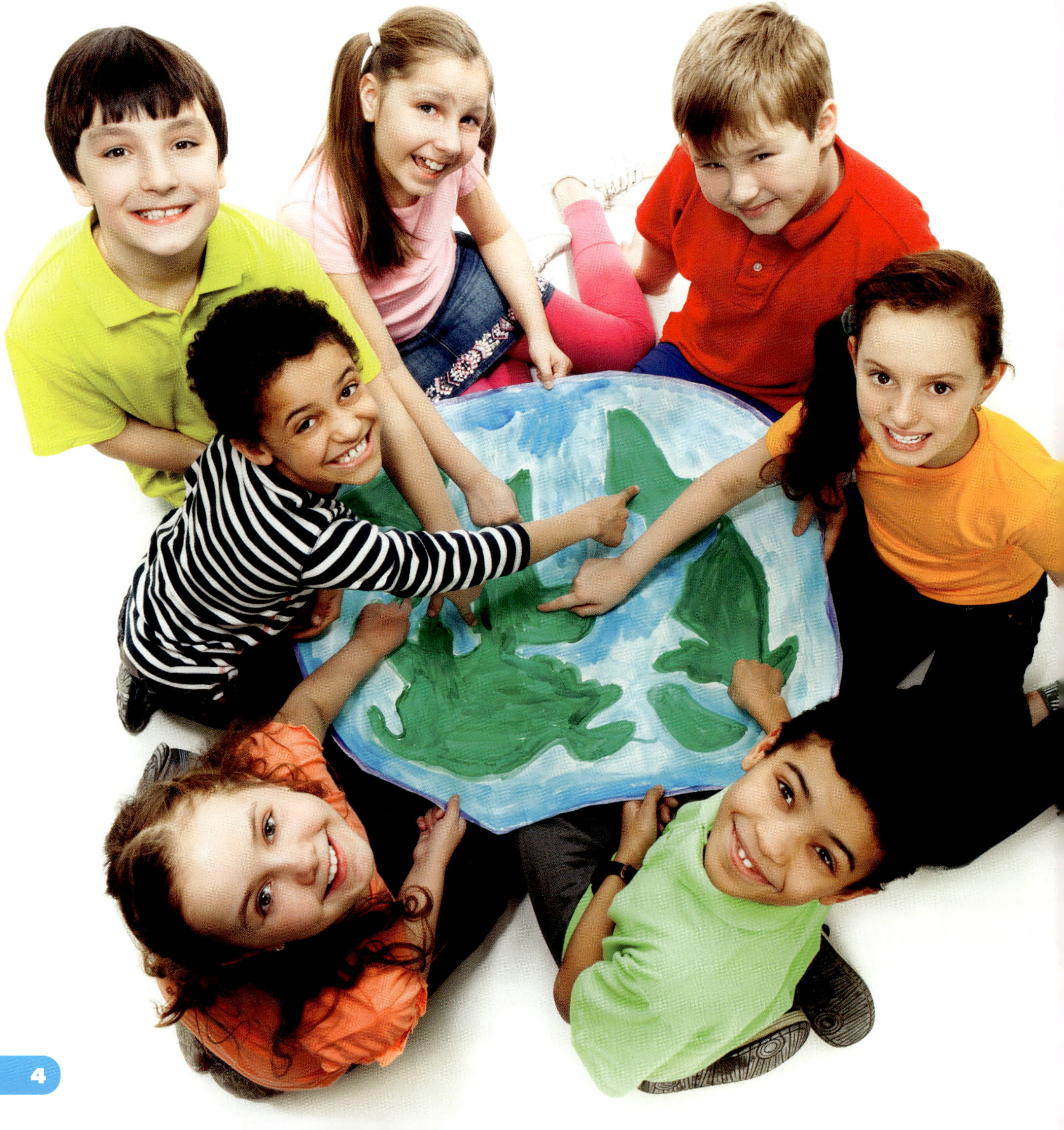

MY BODY AND ME

My Bright Eyes

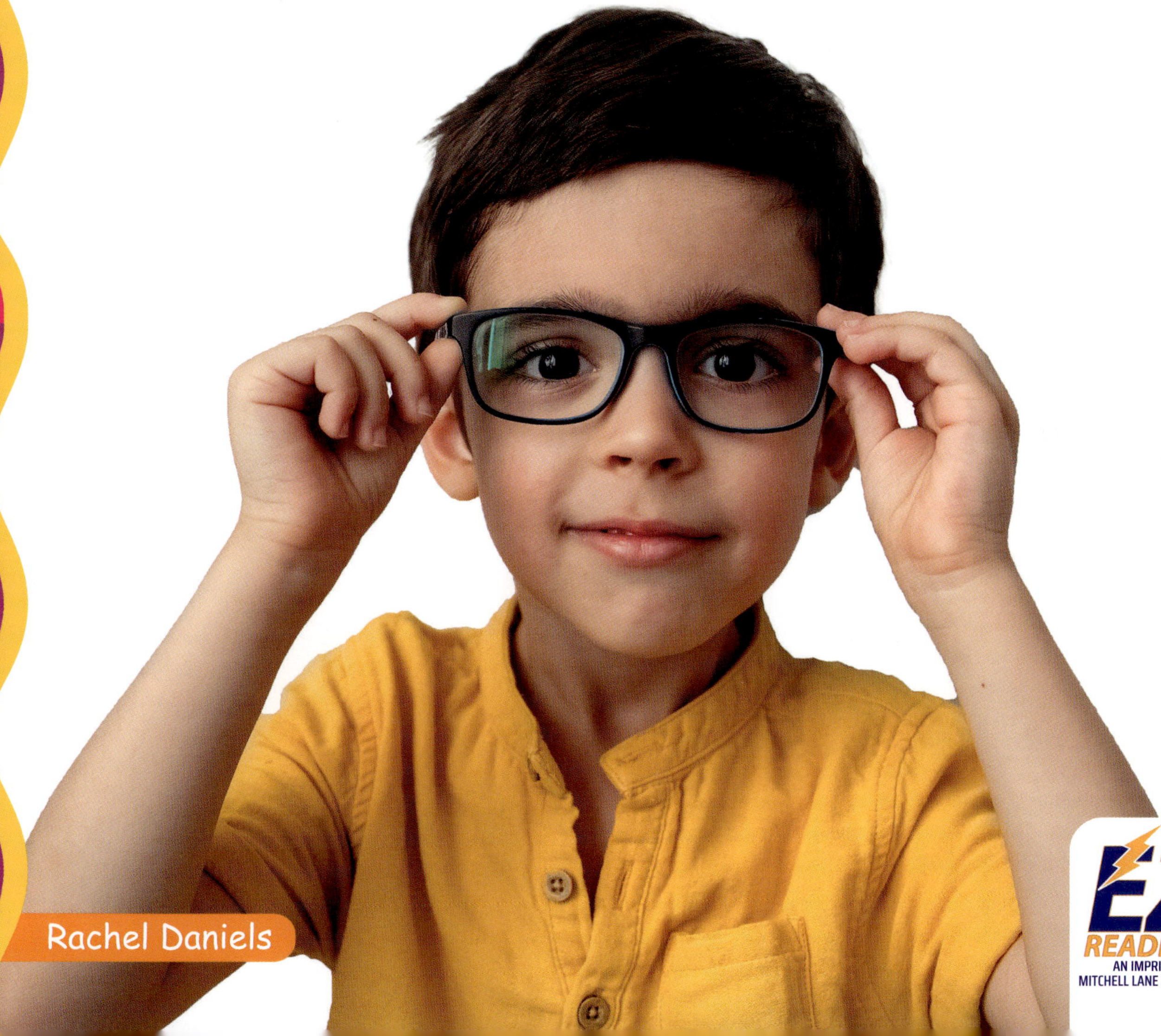

Rachel Daniels

EZ READERS
AN IMPRINT OF
MITCHELL LANE PUBLISHERS

CREATING YOUNG NONFICTION READERS

EZ Readers offer nonfiction for beginning readers in PreK through first grade, using simple language, clear illustrations, and engaging facts to build vocabulary and confidence.

TIPS FOR READING NONFICTION WITH BEGINNING READERS

Talk about Nonfiction

Begin by explaining that nonfiction books give us information that is true. The book will be organized around a specific topic or idea, and we may learn new facts through reading.

Look at the Parts

Most nonfiction books have helpful features. Our *EZ Readers* include color photographs and graphic aids, a table of contents, a glossary, and an index. Share the purpose of these features with your reader.

Color Photos and Graphic Aids

A lot of information can be found by "reading" photos, charts, maps, and other graphic aids found within nonfiction texts. Help your reader learn more about the different ways information can be displayed.

Table of Contents

Located at the front of the book, this list shows the big ideas within the text and the page numbers where they can be found.

Glossary

Located at the back of the book, the glossary defines key words and phrases that are related to the topic. These words and phrases can be found in the text in colored type.

Index

Located at the back of the book, an index is an alphabetical list of topics and the page numbers where they can be found.

With a little help and guidance about reading nonfiction, you can feel good about introducing a young reader to the world of *EZ Readers* nonfiction books.

EZ Readers is an imprint of:

Mitchell Lane PUBLISHERS

2001 SW 31st Avenue
Hallandale, FL 33009
mitchelllanepub.com

First Edition, 2026.

Author: Rachel Daniels
Editor: Morgan Brody

ISBN 979-8-89260-825-1 (library binding)
ISBN 979-8-90145-031-4 (paperback)
ISBN 979-8-89260-834-3 (ebook)

LC record available at https://lccn.loc.gov/2025950823

Photo credits: Shutterstock, Alex Konon, cover, 1, 2, 3, 5, 10, 14, 17, 18, 21; Shutterstock, yusuf_demirci, cover, 1; iStock, Viktoriia Lykhonosova, cover, 1; Shutterstock, Sergey Novikov, 4, 22; iStock, ferrantraite, 7; Shutterstock, Mariia Masich, 8–9; Shutterstock, LuckyStep, 11, 22; Shutterstock, EvGavrilov, 12–13, 22; Shutterstock, Roman Samborskyi, 15, 22; Shutterstock, Andrey Sayfutdinov, 16; iStock, Ridofranz, 19, 22; Shutterstock, LeManna, 20, 22

Look at Me!

My bright eyes open wide.
They help me see the **world**.

Eyes are on my face.

I have two eyes.

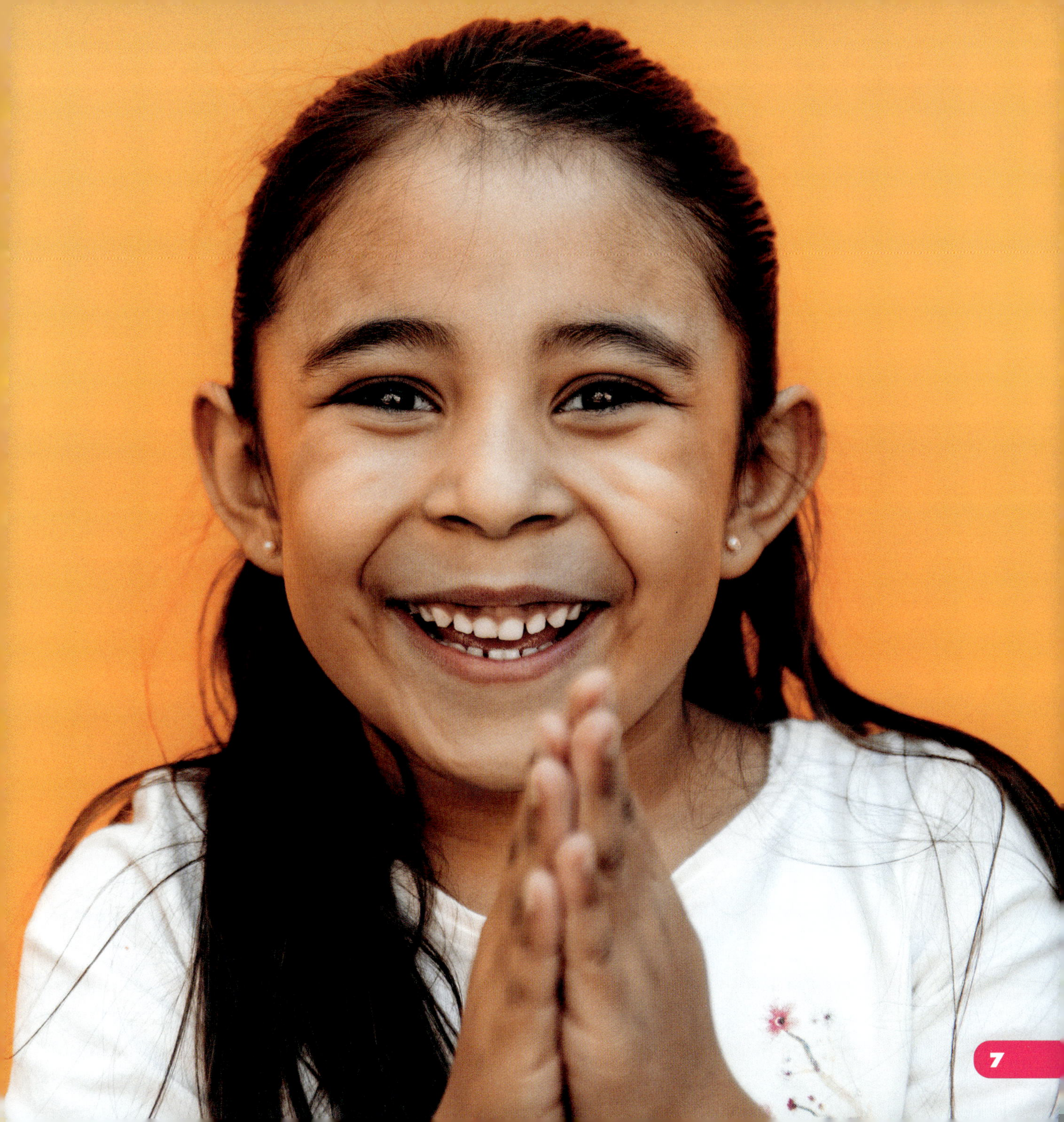

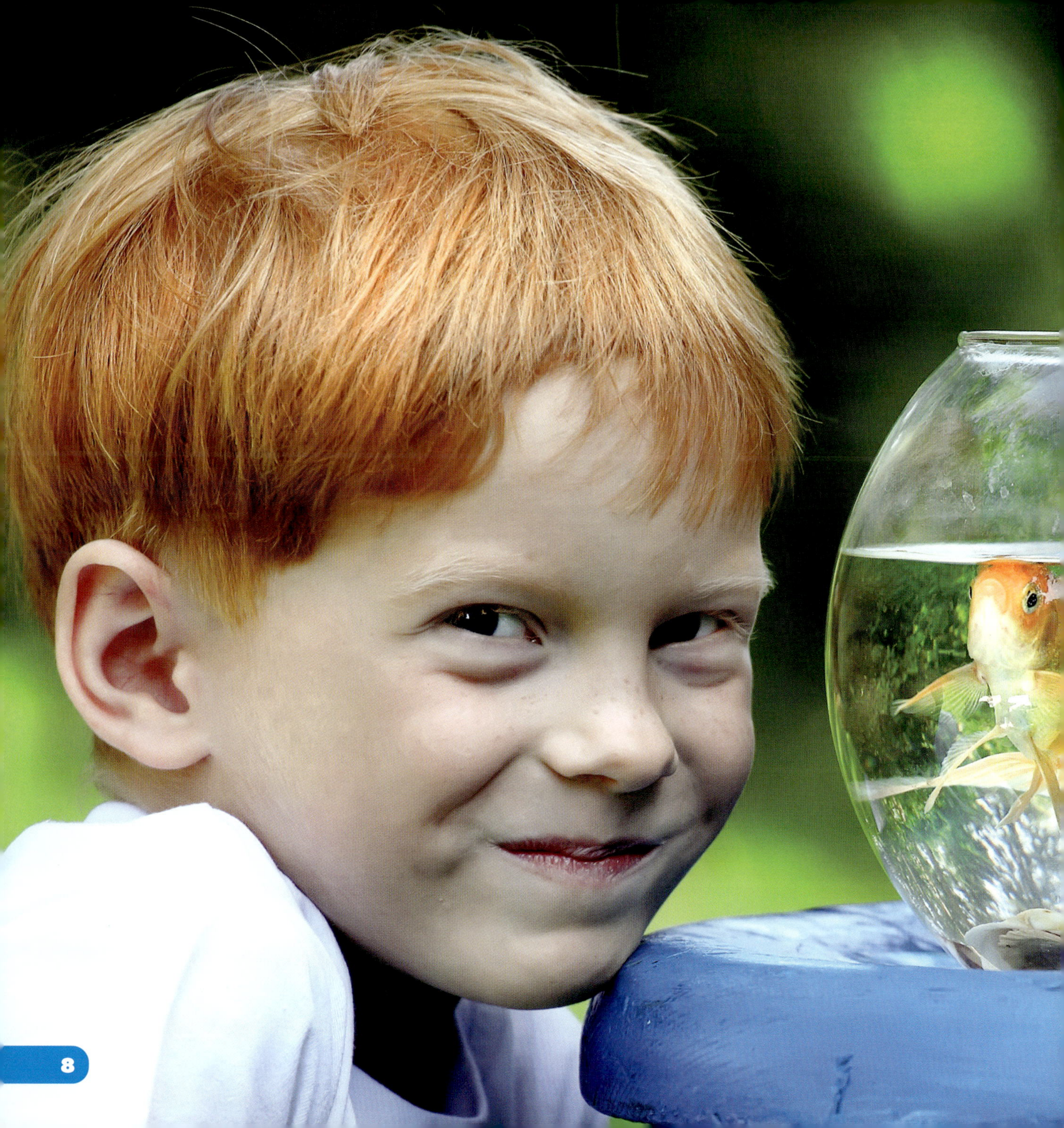

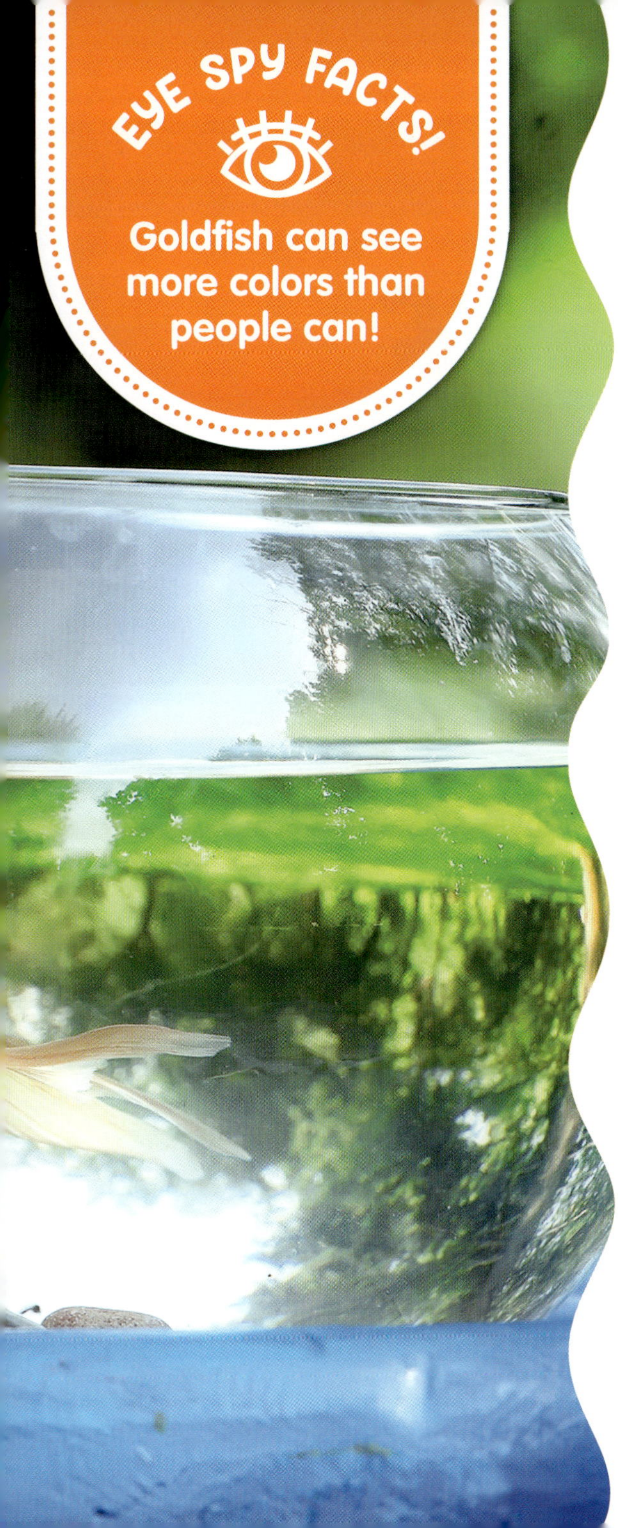

EYE SPY FACTS!

Goldfish can see more colors than people can!

Eyes see light, shapes, and colors.

They help me read and play.

Parts of the Eye

The colored circle is the **iris**.

It makes my eyes brown, blue, or green.

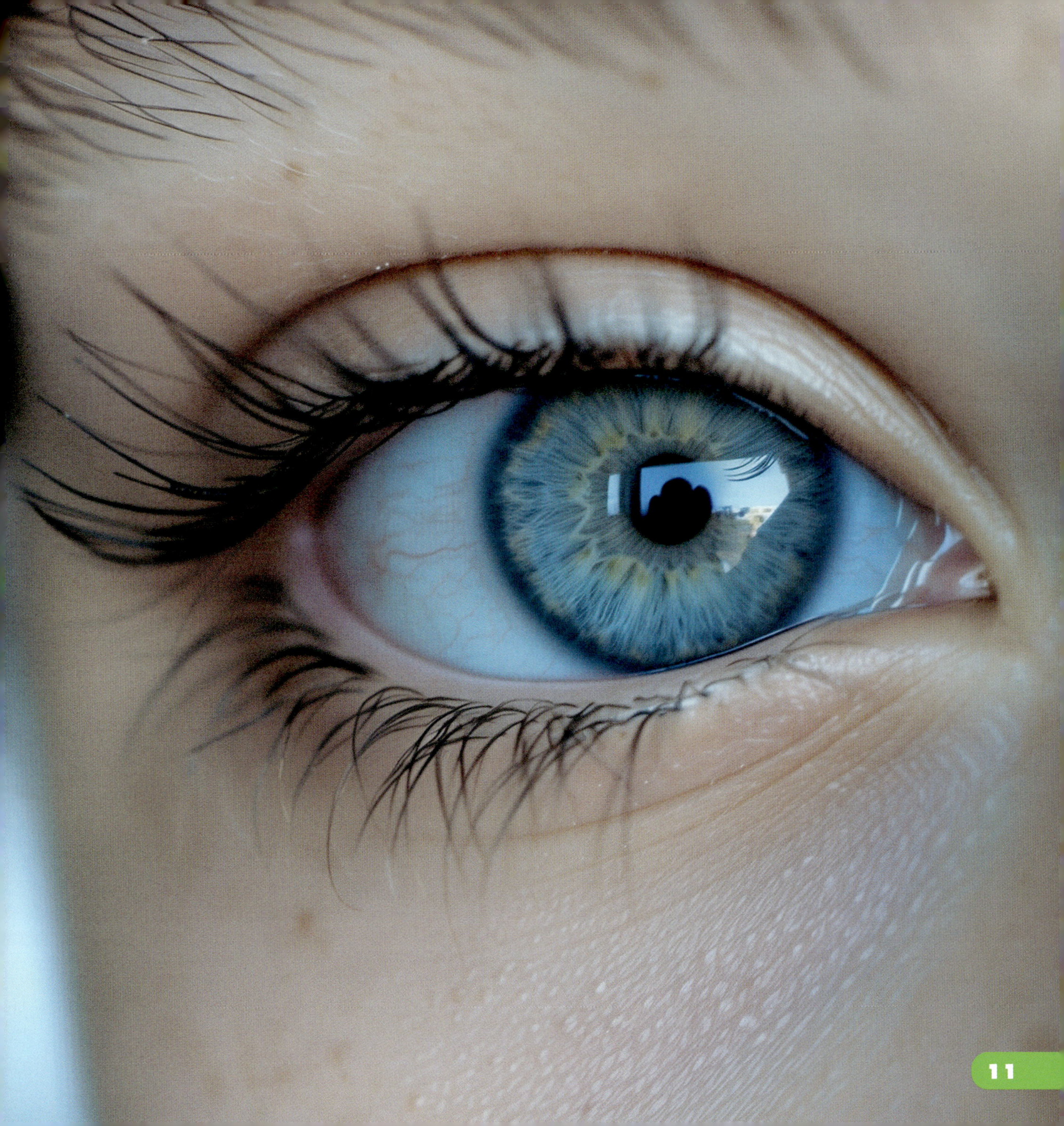

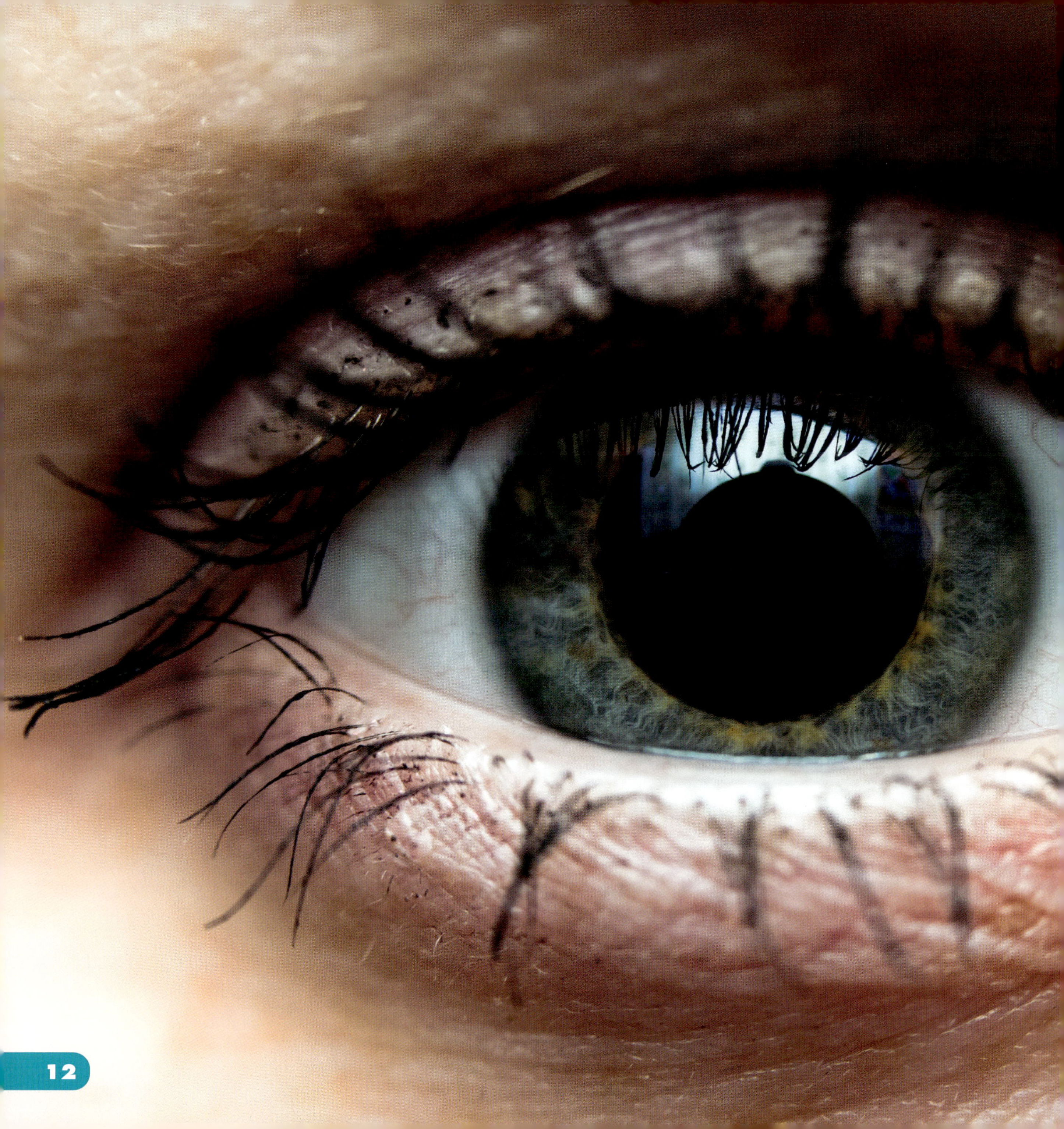

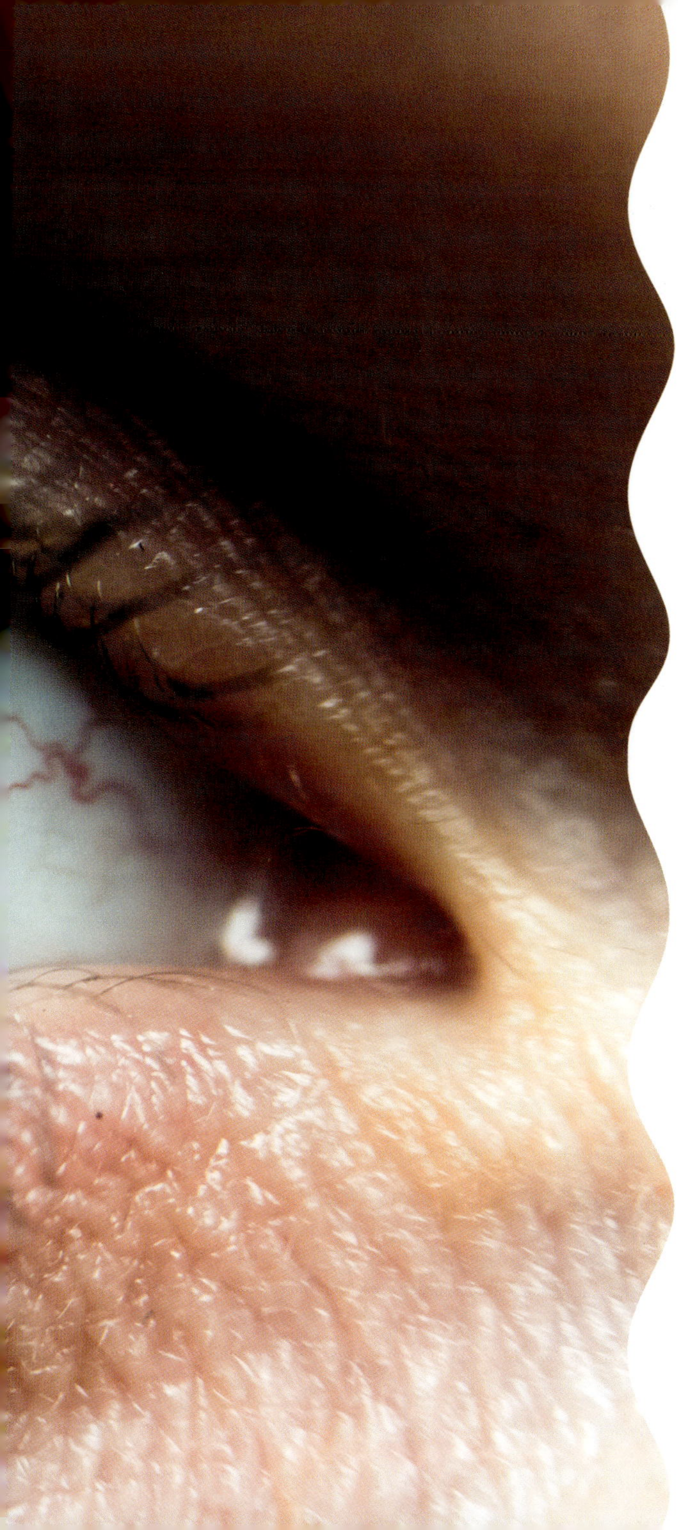

The black dot is the **pupil**.

It gets bigger in the dark.

Blink!

Eyelids blink to keep
eyes safe.

Blink, blink—about
15 times each minute!

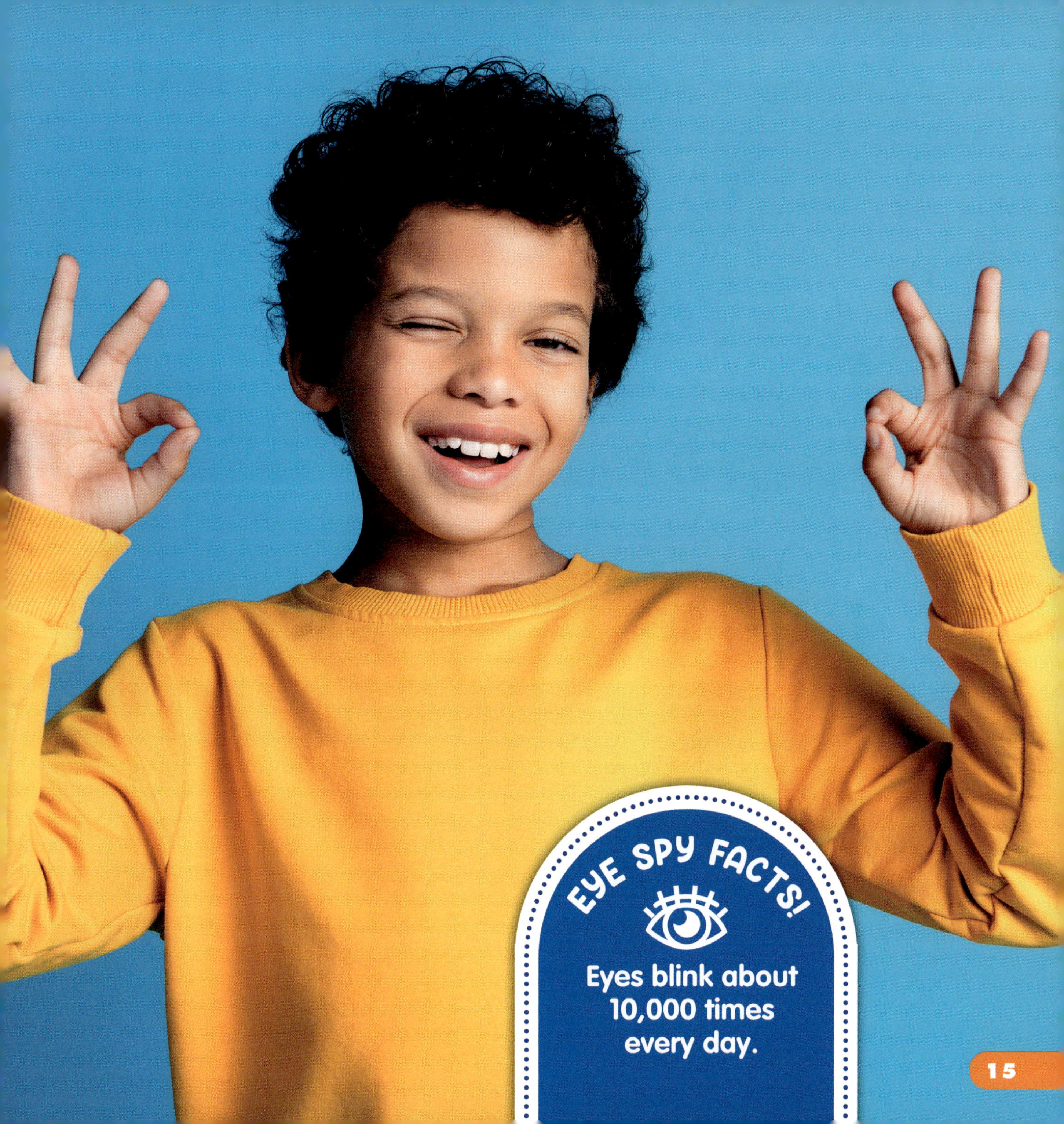

EYE SPY FACTS!

Eyes blink about 10,000 times every day.

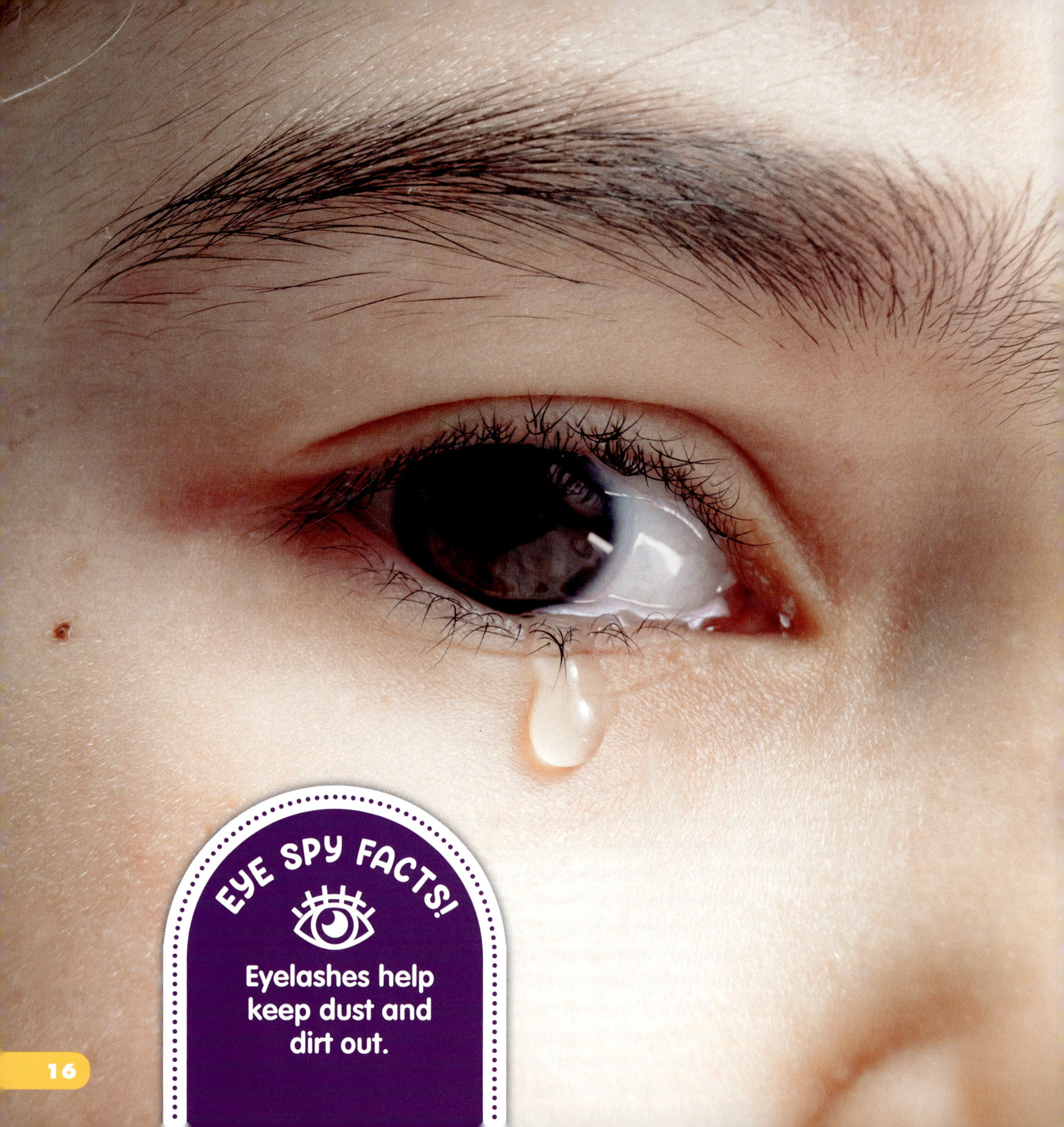

EYE SPY FACTS!

Eyelashes help keep dust and dirt out.

Tears

Tears wash dust away.

They keep eyes
healthy and wet.

Glasses

Some kids wear **glasses**.

Glasses help eyes see clearly.

EYE SPY FACTS!

Owls can see well at night, but people can't.

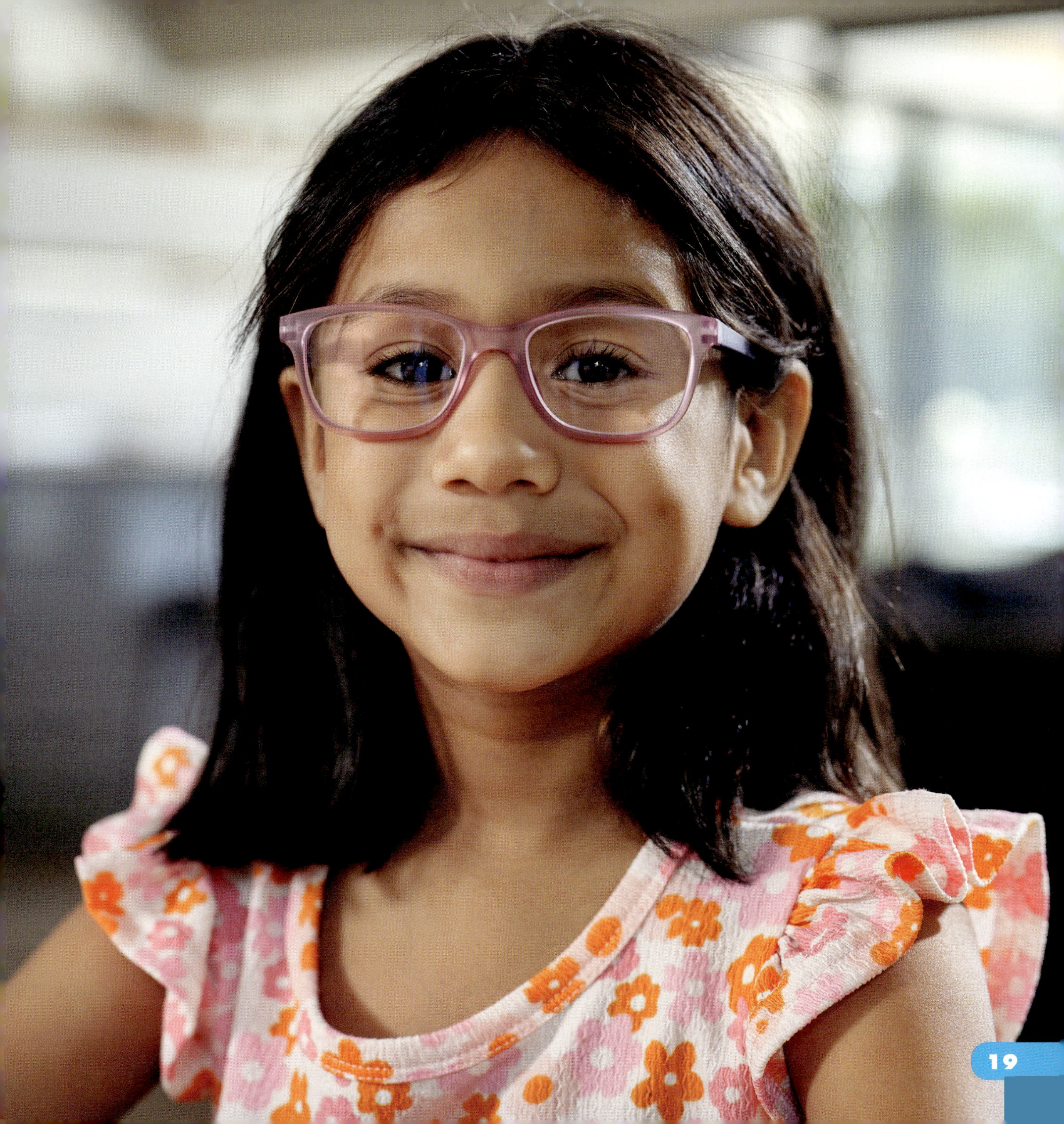

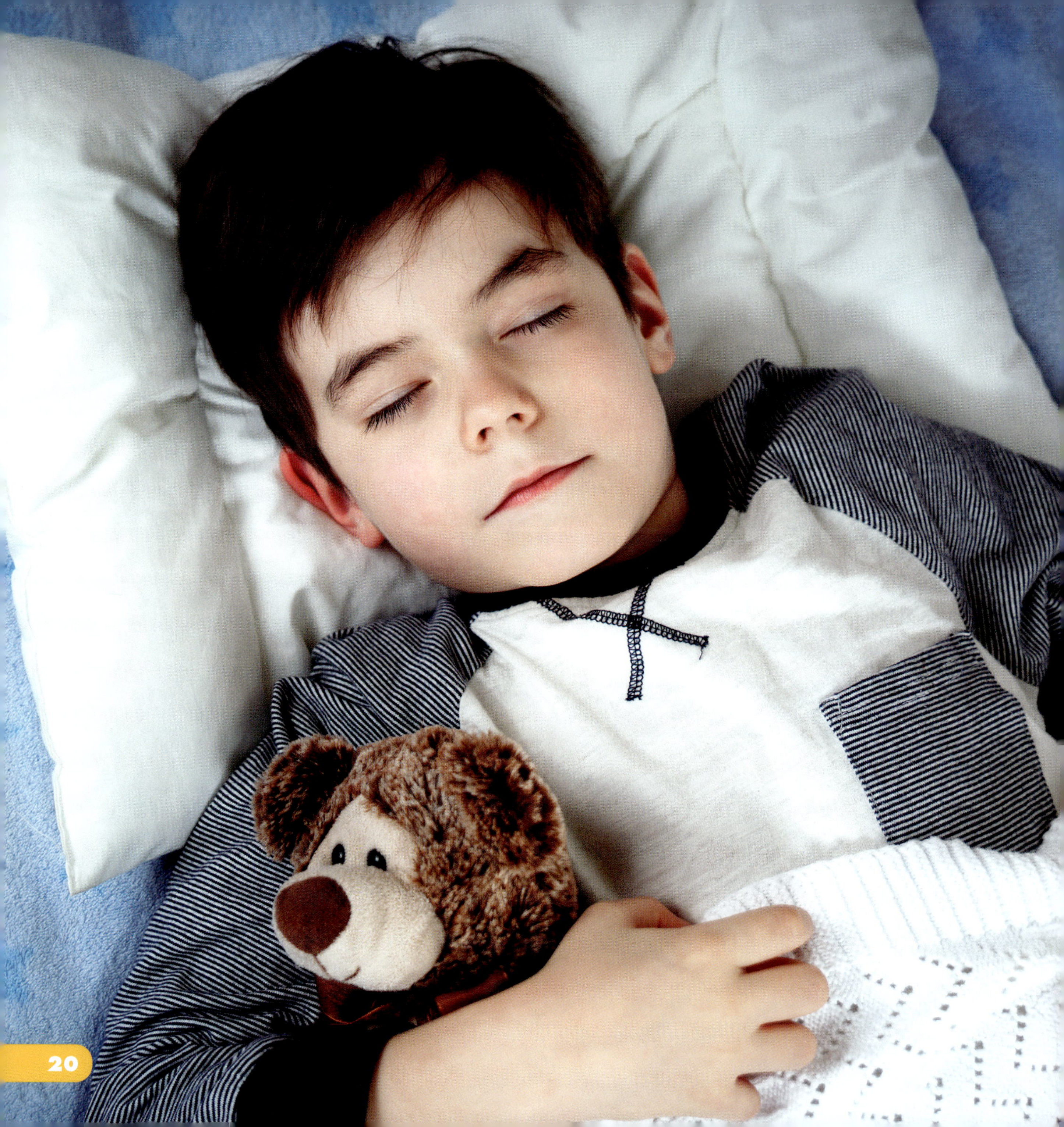

Good Night

Eyes close for sleep.

Tomorrow, my bright eyes will see more!

Glossary

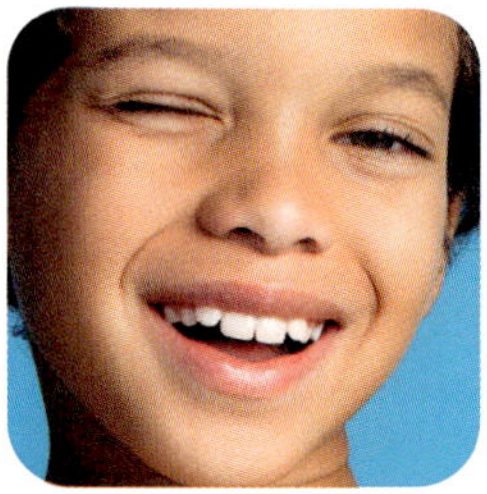

blink (blĭngk) to quickly open and close your eyes

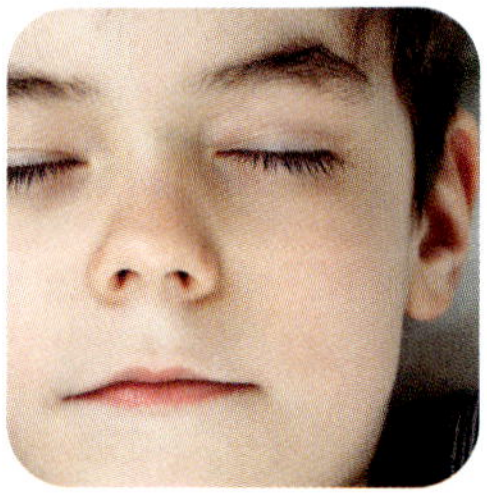

eyelids (EYE-lids) the thin skin that opens and closes over your eyes to protect them

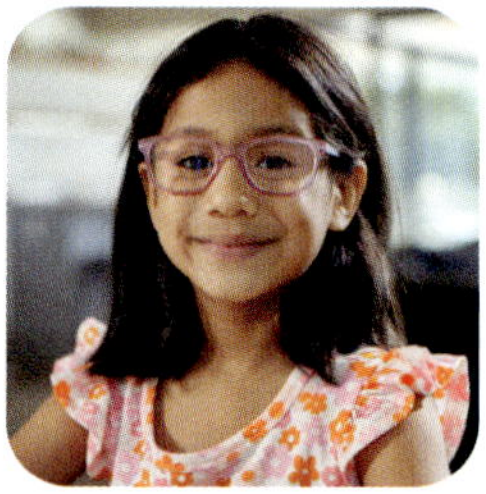

glasses (GLAS-iz) something you wear on your face to help your eyes see better

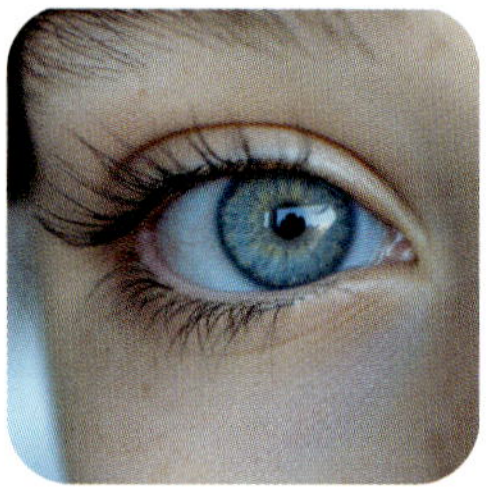

iris (EYE-ris) the colored part of your eye, like blue, brown, or green

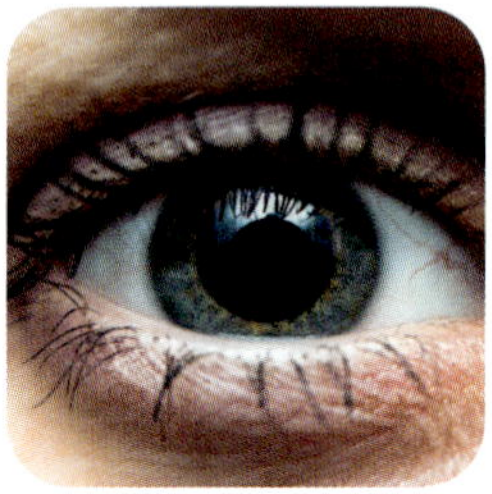

pupil (PYOO-pul) the black dot in the middle of your eye that lets in light

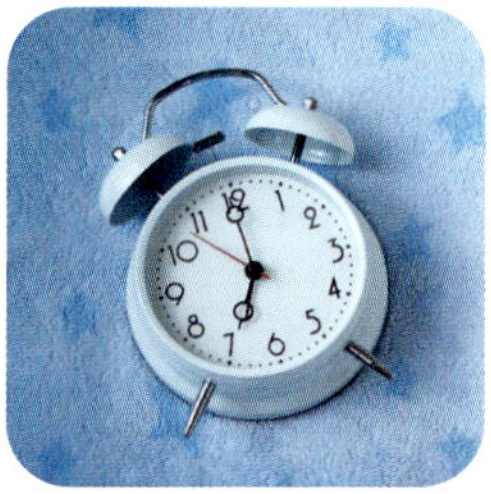

tomorrow (tuh-MAWR-oh) the day that comes after today

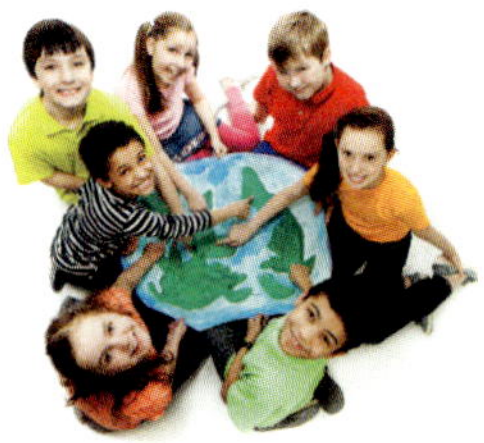

world (WURLD) the Earth, where we all live

Quiz: My Healthy Bones

1. Most people have two eyes.

A. Yes B. No

2. Pupils get bigger in the dark.

A. Yes B. No

3. Tears keep your eyes healthy and wet.

A. Yes B. No

4. Glasses help people see clearly.

A. Yes B. No

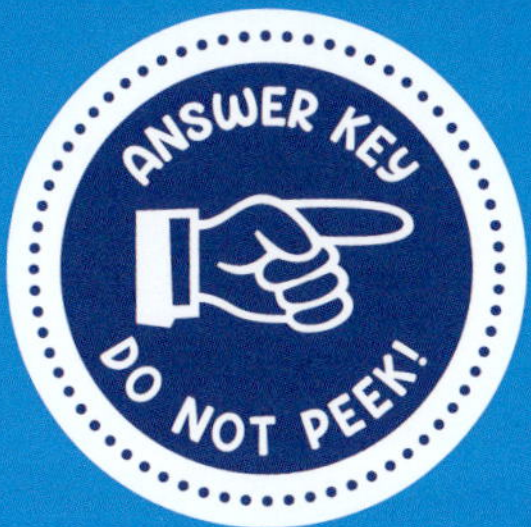

ANSWER KEY:

How many times did you answer yes?

4 Yes: Awesome! You know your eyes well.

3 Yes: Great! You learned some new facts.

2 Yes: That's okay! Keep reading.

1 Yes: You're starting to learn. Keep going!

Further Reading

Culliford, Amy. *My Body Has Eyes.* Crabtree. 2022.

Rose, Rachel. *I Need an Eye Doctor.* Bearport Publishing, 2025.

On the Internet

Britannica Kids: Eye

https://kids.britannica.com/kids/article/eye/353116

A brief, age-appropriate article with simple sentences and fun facts like how eyelids blink and tears keep eyes moist.

KidsHealth—Your Eyes

https://kidshealth.org/en/kids/eyes.html

A child-friendly page that explains what eyes do, how they work, and fun facts.

Index

About the Author

Rachel Daniels is a former elementary school teacher who loves reading and discovering new things. She lives in sunny South Florida with her husband, close to her children and grandchildren. When she's not reading or writing, she enjoys playing Canasta with friends. Her goal is to make learning exciting and joyful for young readers everywhere.